IMPROVING HIGH BLOOD PRESSURE IN 30 DAYS

Hypertension and Hypotension Relief within 30
Days, Blood Pressure Recovery Plan
for Long-Term Health

By Robert Redfern

About the Author

Your Personal Health Coach
www.MyGoodHealthClub.com

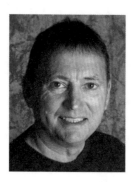

Robert Redfern (born January 1946) has helped hundreds of thousands of people in over 24 countries through online health support websites, books, radio/TV interviews, and his nutritional discoveries. His new series of books brings this work together in an easy-to-read format that everyone can follow to help resolve their chronic health problem – once and for all.

Robert's interest in health started when he and his wife Anne decided to take charge of their family's health in the late 1980s. Up until 1986, Robert had not taken much notice of his health – in spite of Anne's loving persuasion. It took the premature death of his parents, Alfred and Marjorie, who died in their sixties, to shock Robert into evaluating his priorities.

Robert and Anne looked at the whole field of health, available treatments and the causes of health problems. They found, from doctors researching the causes of disease, that lifestyle and diet were the most important contributions to health. Robert and Anne changed their lifestyle and diet and, together with the use of **HealthPoint™** acupressure, the improvement to their health was remarkable.

▸ *As well as good health, they feel and look younger and more energetic than all those years ago – before they started their plan. At the time of printing, Robert, aged 68, and Anne have every intention of continuing to be well and looking younger, using their unique understanding of Natural Health.* ◂

ROBERT REDFERN - YOUR PERSONAL HEALTH COACH
tells you everything you need to know about:

High Blood Pressure (Hypertension) & Low Blood Pressure (Hypotension)

Using the Science and Knowledge of a Non-Inflammatory Lifestyle to Achieve Healthy Blood Pressure

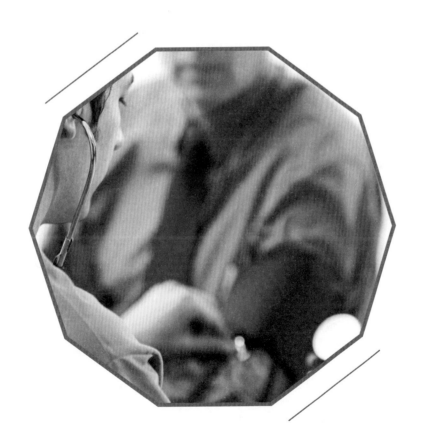

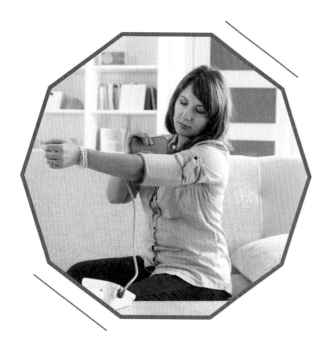

Publisher:

Naturally Healthy Publications. All rights reserved.

Reader is not permitted to reproduce any part of this book without obtaining written permission from the author.

Publication printed in the United Kingdom.

Publisher's Note:

This book is not intended to diagnose any disease or offer medical advice. The intention of the book is only to provide information for the reader so that they can make healthy lifestyle choices.

Warning:

Some of the information in this book may contradict advice from your physician; nonetheless, content is based on the science of natural health.

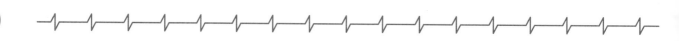

CONTENTS

YOUR ACTION PLAN TO COMMIT TO A NON-INFLAMMATORY LIFESTYLE TO ACHIEVE HEALTHY BLOOD PRESSURE

TODAY	I DID THIS	SIGNED	DATE
I Committed	To regaining and maintaining a non-inflammatory lifestyle for the rest of my life		
I Committed	To drinking 6-8 glasses of water a day		
I Committed	To getting out in the sun for 20 minutes a day (except when contraindicated)		
I Read	Robert's Healthy Blood Pressure Book		
I Ordered	The necessary supplements to facilitate my plan and my healing		
I Planned	My Daily Menu with **ReallyHealthyFoods.com**		
I Started	My breathing exercises		
I Started	Massaging the acupressure points		
I Reread	Robert's Healthy Blood Pressure Book		
I Reviewed	The necessary supplements to facilitate my plan and my healing		
I Reviewed	My water intake		
I Reviewed	My menu		
I Reviewed	My breathing exercises		
I Reviewed	My life-giving sun exposure (except when contraindicated)		
I Reviewed	Massaging the acupressure points		
I Recommitted	To regaining and maintaining a non-inflammatory lifestyle		
I Recommitted	To Robert's Healthy Blood Pressure Book		
I Recommitted	To taking the necessary supplements to facilitate a non-inflammatory lifestyle		
I Recommitted	To my water intake		
I Recommitted	To following my menu		
I Recommitted	To doing my breathing exercises		
I Recommitted	To life-giving sun exposure (except when contraindicated)		
I Recommitted	To massaging the acupressure points		

1. What Is Blood Pressure?

Blood pressure is the force required to maintain the blood flow throughout the body. Blood pressure can be further defined as the blood in the body exerting force (pressure) against the artery walls while the heart is pumping blood.

High Blood Pressure

High blood pressure is when force is too high. High blood pressure is very common and can be life-threatening when blood pressure is consistently <u>above what is considered healthy.</u> It can lead to many other serious conditions, including cardiovascular disease. High blood pressure is a major factor in damaging the blood vessels, a precursor to having a stroke.

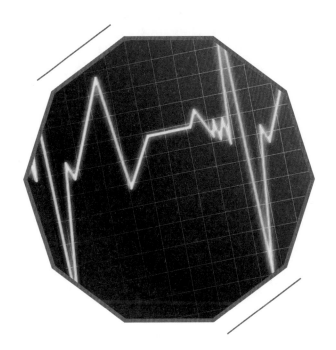

*   **High blood pressure/hypertension** is when blood pressure is consistently high.

*   **Low blood pressure/hypotension** is when blood pressure is consistently low.

> ▸ *Both of these conditions, especially hypertension, can be signs of underlying health problems and are potentially dangerous to the body.* ◂

The Heart

The heart is a muscular pump (technically, a circulator) and plays a crucial role in the circulatory system. It's the hardest working muscle we have as it works non-stop, 24 hours a day, making its ability to function at an optimum level that much more important.

> ▸ *The heart is approximately the size of your fist and is located underneath the ribs, slightly to the left of the center of the chest.* ◂

As a circulator, the heart can only work effectively as part of the entire healthy, active circulatory system acting in unison. The circulatory system is composed of muscles, veins, arteries, and joints. The blood in your feet can't get back to your heart and lungs without the joints in your legs, feet, and hips moving to aid the circulatory process. The heart could not successfully circulate blood on its own.

When this process is compromised, it leads to damage to the major organs fed by the circulatory system:

A. Heart
B. Kidneys
C. Brain
D. Eyes

The heart and circulatory system's primary purposes are to:

- Circulate oxygen-laden blood and nutrients throughout the body via the arteries.

- Receive and exchange oxygen-poor blood and carbon dioxide from the body, deliver it back to the lungs where it can find fresh oxygen, and pump it back to the heart through the veins.

> ▸ *These purposes are clearly essential to life!* ◂

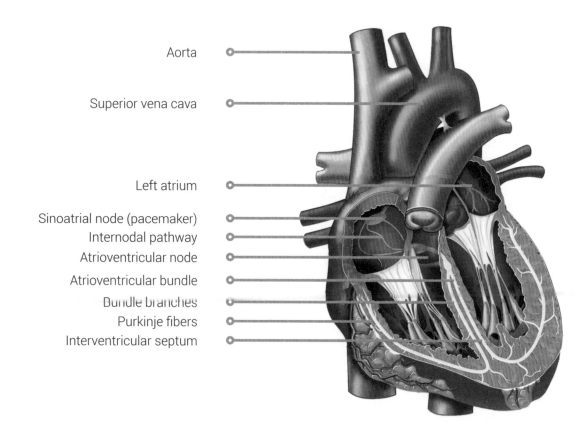

Aorta
Superior vena cava
Left atrium
Sinoatrial node (pacemaker)
Internodal pathway
Atrioventricular node
Atrioventricular bundle
Bundle branches
Purkinje fibers
Interventricular septum

Heart Valves

Certain conditions, including inflammation, hypertension, and cardiovascular disease, can damage the heart valves. The resulting heart valve disease is when one or more valves are dysfunctional due to a change in the shape or flexibility of the valves.

Coronary Arteries

The heart also has its own blood vessels called the coronary arteries.

The three main arteries are:

1. **Right coronary artery (RCA)**
2. **Circumflex artery (CX)**
3. **Left anterior descending artery (LAD)**

When these arteries become diseased, coronary artery disease (CAD) is present. *Keep in mind that hypertension is a primary risk factor for this disease and encourages its development.*

Coronary artery disease is known by a multitude of names or medical terms, including:

- **Hardening of the arteries**
- **Clogged arteries**
- **Plaque build-up**
- **Atherosclerosis**

As we can see, the heart and its ventricles, valves, and arteries, in addition to the rest of the cardiovascular system, are all subject to damage as a result of having high blood pressure.

▸ *This makes hypertension and hypertensive cardiovascular disease grave health concerns.* ◂

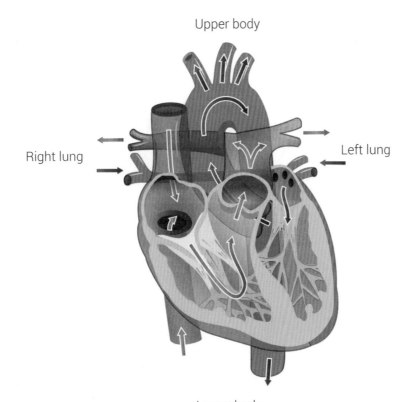

Upper body

Right lung

Left lung

Lower body

2. What Are the Different Types of Blood Pressure?

Hypertension

Hypertension is often thought about in the same way many of us think about diabetes. It's common, part of aging, half the people you know have it, and you just have to live with it! The sad truth is that you can live with high blood pressure for a while. But the reality is that you have a much better chance of dying from complications related to the condition.

The World Health Organization's (WHO) *World Health Statistics 2012* report tells us that hypertension is responsible for approximately half of all deaths that stem from having a stroke or heart disease. These numbers do not include deaths from any other related conditions.

Who Has It?

> ▸ *One in three people across the globe experience high blood pressure.* ◂

Older Age

The incidence of hypertension tends to rise with age. More than 50% of those living in western countries over the age of 60 have hypertension. And worse than that, they have up to a 90% risk of developing high blood pressure over the course of their lives.

Who Has the Highest Risk?

Men and women of black ancestry have the highest risk of getting hypertension. Whether or not this population has a genetic predisposition is debatable; however, what is not up for debate is the substantially higher rate of hypertension in the black community.

Risks can be attributed to:

- Poor diet
- Obesity
- Smoking
- Avoiding exercise
- Taking birth control pills (for women)
- Diabetes
- Drinking too much alcohol
- Undergoing stress in relationships
- Depression

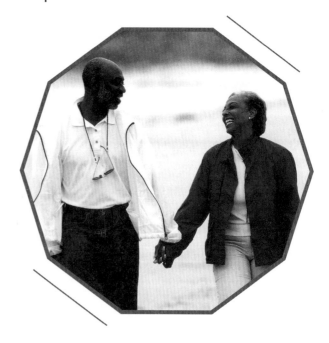

Hypertension Risk Factors

- **Age and Gender** - Men have higher rates of hypertension than women, up to a certain age. Hypertension affects more women after the age of 55 (post-menopause); almost one in three women in the United States has hypertension.

- **Race** - High blood pressure occurs much more often and earlier in the black population than in the white population (30-40% vs. 20%). Black people are also more susceptible to the complications associated with high blood pressure, e.g. heart attack and stroke.

- **Weight** - Being obese or even just a few pounds above a healthy weight means your body requires more blood to do the same job. When there is more blood traveling through your blood vessels, it creates more pressure on the walls of the arteries.

- **Lack of Exercise** - Exercise lowers the heart rate, decreases the number of times the heart beats, and leads to less pressure on the artery walls. It's also easier to maintain a healthy weight when physically active.

- **Tobacco Use** - Any tobacco use (exposure to second-hand smoke, smoking, chewing tobacco) will increase blood pressure in the short-term. Long-term, it will cause narrowing of the arteries, a predecessor to high blood pressure.

- **Excessive Salt Compared to Potassium** - Sodium beyond what your body needs for potassium balance can raise blood pressure; too little potassium can equate to too much sodium.

- **Vitamin D3 Deficiency** - Vitamin D may influence an enzyme manufactured by the kidneys that alters blood pressure. Several studies have shown a positive correlation.

- **Alcohol** - Excessive drinking can be detrimental to the heart; just three drinks a day or more can elevate blood pressure.

- **Poor Breathing and Anxiety** - Both can raise blood pressure.

- **Certain Medications** – This includes corticosteroids, NSAIDs, antihistamines, weight loss pills, birth control pills, and some types of antidepressants.

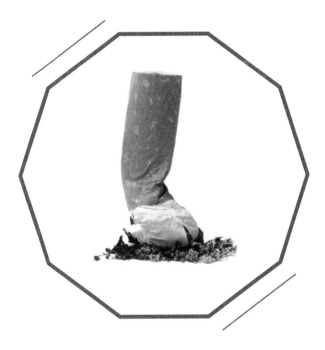

Hypertension and Inflammation

An anti-inflammatory approach to diet, in addition to making other healthy lifestyle choices, will at a minimum lower blood pressure, if not completely eliminate hypertension in most cases.

This approach includes the following foods:

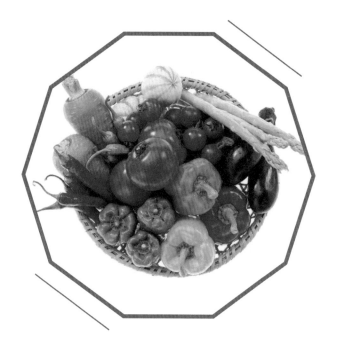

- Any kind of vegetables, focusing on non-starchy vegetables, especially dark leafy greens; yams/ sweet potatoes are fine in moderation.

- Legumes; beans, peas, and lentils of all kinds.

- Alternative to grains and cereals; Quinoa, millet, buckwheat, and other seeds.

- Low sugar, dark-skinned fruits like avocados, blueberries, blackberries, black currants, etc.

- Hemp seeds daily.

Here are a few more important tips to remember about high blood pressure and diet:

- An inadequate intake of vitamin C has been associated with higher blood pressure; 500 or more mg of vitamin C a day has been associated with lower blood pressure (*Advances in Pharmacological Sciences,* Volume 2011).

- A diet low in or completely devoid of meat may have the potential to lower blood pressure as saturated fat (high in animal products) seems to affect the viscosity (thickness) of the blood. Blood viscosity, according to research, is higher in those with hypertension.

We will discuss high blood pressure rehabilitation through dietary changes further on **page 28.**

Hypertension and Cardiovascular Disease

Most of the risk factors for hypertension are simply unhealthy choices, which are part of an inflammatory lifestyle. The resulting high blood pressure is then a primary risk factor for many other chronic conditions and diseases, especially cardiovascular disease.

When looking at cardiovascular disease, specifically, coronary artery disease, we find it is the number one cause of death in the United States. The majority of these deaths stem from heart attacks as a result of unexpected blood clots in the arteries.

▸ *How does hypertension contribute to this deadly disease?* ◂

The added pressure against the walls of the arteries damages the arteries. When the integrity of the arteries is compromised, they become more susceptible to the constriction and build-up of plaque associated with atherosclerosis. This reduces or completely blocks blood flow to the heart, limiting the amount of oxygen the heart receives. This process is exactly what precedes a cardiovascular incident.

What Is Hypertensive Cardiovascular Disease?

Hypertensive cardiovascular disease refers to cardiovascular problems that occur because of high blood pressure.

▸ *Hypertensive cardiovascular disease is the number one cause of death stemming from high blood pressure.* ◂

What Causes Hypertension and Hypertensive Cardiovascular Disease?

▸ *Simply an inflammatory, unnatural lifestyle.* ◂

Too much cholesterol, right? Not necessarily! Cholesterol is actually essential for good health. The liver produces enough cholesterol every day to provide a healthy level of hormones, support brain function, and protect and defend the body against inflammation.

While cholesterol is definitely beneficial to the body, **oxidized cholesterol** is one of the culprits responsible for progressing cardiovascular disease. Cholesterol becomes oxidized when it is exposed to free radicals (unstable and highly reactive molecules that wreak havoc in the body). Oxidized cholesterol has the ability to enter cells in excess, contributing to the damage (inflammation) already present in the arteries.

While we need some level of free radicals to function - and it's not possible to eliminate them completely - most of us have way too many. Fortunately, antioxidants, available in high quality foods and supplements, can fight off these free radicals and the damage they do to the body. Good sources are beans, berries, and other fruits and vegetables.

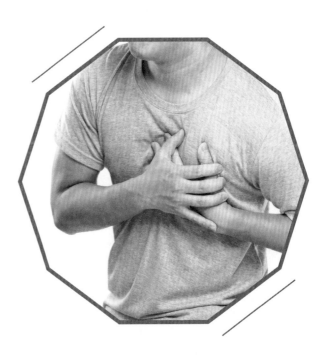

Non-Inflammatory Solutions for Hypertension and Hypertensive Cardiovascular Disease

Fortunately, the things we need to do (or not do) to prevent hypertension and hypertensive cardiovascular diseases are the same. <u>They are all part of a non-inflammatory, healthy lifestyle.</u>

Yet based on the numbers associated with these conditions, most of us are not embracing this lifestyle.

A non-inflammatory, healthy lifestyle directed toward preventing or correcting hypertension and hypertensive cardiovascular disease includes:

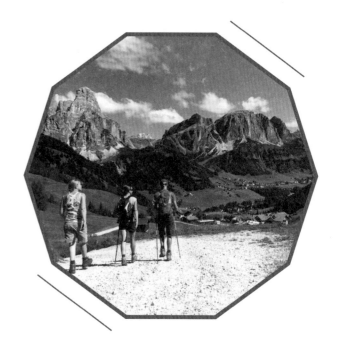

- Maintaining a healthy weight
- Exercising regularly
- Avoiding tobacco use of any kind
- Minimizing processed salt intake
- Increasing potassium intake
- Getting enough vitamin D3
- Limiting alcohol (one drink a day for women, two for men)
- Relieving stress
- Looking for alternatives to medication

Hypotension

Although the focus of this book has been on high blood pressure, hypotension or abnormally low blood pressure is of concern to those who struggle with it. This is because hypotension results in the brain not getting what it needs, i.e. not receiving enough blood, or more importantly, the oxygen within that blood.

There seem to be no solid numbers on how many people experience low blood pressure as the condition can be temporary or situational. It is estimated that 10-20% of those over 65 have a certain type of hypotension referred to as postural hypotension.

Hypotension is usually diagnosed when pressure is 90/60 and accompanied by symptoms, like:

- Dizziness
- Light-headedness
- Fainting
- Dehydration
- Inability to concentrate
- Compromised vision
- Nausea
- Cold, clammy, pale skin
- Fast chest breathing
- Extreme tiredness
- Depression
- Thirst

Much of the time, there's no need to be alarmed about having low blood pressure. Mild symptoms may be perfectly fine. Certain individuals have a naturally low, naturally healthy blood pressure.

These individuals are:

- Physically fit
- At a healthy weight
- Eating a healthy diet
- Non-smokers

There are positive consequences to having low blood pressure, including a lower incidence of:

- Stroke
- Kidney disease
- Heart disease

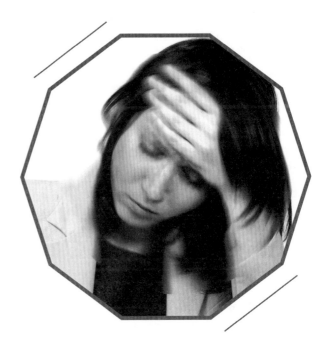

Hypotension Risk Factors

Although hypotension is not exclusive to any one group, there are certain risk factors associated with this condition: Yet based on the numbers associated with these conditions, most of us are not embracing this lifestyle.

- **Stage of Life** - Depending upon the type of hypotension, it can affect seniors, kids, and younger adults.

- **Other Conditions and Diseases** - Parkinson's disease, diabetes, and a few heart conditions can put you at a higher risk for hypotension.

- **Prescription Drugs** - Some drugs taken for hypertension can lead to hypotension.

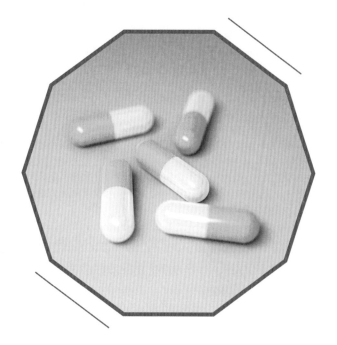

As we know, drugs come with many side effects and can be quite dangerous, especially for the older population. Calcium channel blockers and beta blockers may decrease the amount of time it takes for the heart to contract, leading to an extremely slow heart rate.

These drugs can also, along with ACE inhibitors, angiotensin receptor blockers, alpha-blockers, and diuretics, decrease blood pressure so significantly that symptoms can start to appear.

Drugs used for the following conditions can also lower blood pressure:

- **Parkinson's disease**
- **Depression**
- **Sexual dysfunction**

Drinking alcohol and taking illegal drugs can lead to hypotension.

Hypotension and Inflammation

Inflammation as a result of lifestyle choices has many implications when it comes to hypertension. *Does the same apply to hypotension?*

A prime example of hypotension stemming from inflammation can be found with extreme inflammation of various organs. The pancreas is one such organ. A diagnosis of acute pancreatitis comes from discovering fluid is pooling around the tissues that surround the pancreas and abdominal area, leaving a concentration of blood and a decreased blood volume.

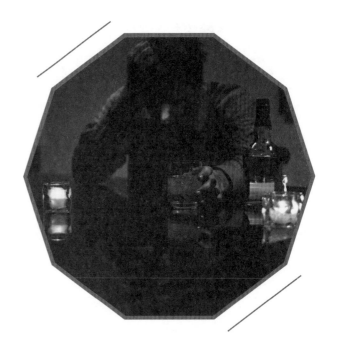

Another form of inflammation resulting in low blood pressure is pericarditis. Pericarditis is inflammation of the sac encircling the heart. It is responsible for fluid gathering within the sac and crushing the heart, limiting the heart's ability to function properly.

Inflammatory conditions or lifestyle choices associated with hypotension include:

- Heart disease/complications
- Nutritional deficiencies
- Alcohol use
- Drug use
- Dehydration
- Adrenal gland dysfunction

We have discussed most of these already in regards to an inflammatory lifestyle, with the exception of adrenal gland dysfunction. Adrenal gland dysfunction stems primarily from too much stress.

It is also greatly affected by the Western Unnatural Food Diet and other factors associated with an unhealthy lifestyle, like:

- Smoking
- Alcohol abuse
- Lack of sleep
- Drugs
- Caffeine
- Too much or too little exercise

Do any of these sound familiar?

Conditions That Cause Low Blood Pressure

- **Being Pregnant** - Causes the circulatory system to extend at a faster rate, meaning less blood is available to do the same job. It's natural during the first six months of pregnancy for pressure to decrease and should normalize again after giving birth.

- **Heart Conditions** - A previous heart attack, heart failure, prescription drugs, viral infections, or heart valve disease may decrease the volume of blood the heart pumps.

- **Endocrine Concerns** – May involve the thyroid, either from being too active (hyperthyroidism) or not active enough (hypothyroidism); the adrenal glands (adrenal gland fatigue, Addison's disease); low blood sugar (hypoglycemia); and, in certain circumstances, diabetes.

- **Adrenal Gland** - Dysfunction results in adrenal gland fatigue, a condition in which the adrenal glands are not fully functioning. The adrenal glands are responsible for a myriad of bodily functions, including the regulation of blood pressure, the release of stress hormones, and the functioning of the heart.

- **Dehydration** - When the body is in a negative water balance, it can cause symptoms like light-headedness, tiredness, weakness, and even hypovolemic shock, resulting in organ failure. Dehydration may be caused by fever, vomiting, diarrhea, excessive diuretic use, and too much exercise.

- **Losing Blood** - In excessive amounts.

- **Septic Shock** - From a harsh infection invading the blood.

- **Anaphylactic Shock** - A severe allergic reaction to food, medications, and insect bites that can end in death. Reactions include hives, wheezing, a swollen throat, and difficulty breathing.

- **Nutritional Deficiencies** - Can lead to anemia, a condition in which the body is incapable of making an adequate amount of red blood cells. B-12 and folate are both needed in the proper amounts in order to avoid anemia.

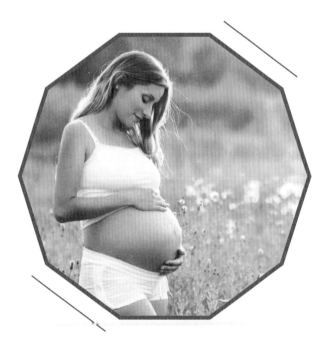

Hypertension, Cardiovascular Disease, and Diabetes

> ▸ *What do hypertension, cardiovascular disease, and diabetes all have in common?* ◂

The connection may be surprising. The leading cause of mortality for those with diabetes *is cardiovascular disease!* We already know that hypertension is a primary risk factor for these diseases.

> ▸ *Hypertension occurs almost twice as often in those suffering from diabetes as opposed to those who do not have this chronic disease.* ◂

If this scenario scares you, the numbers also show that those with high blood pressure are much more likely to develop diabetes than those who avoid hypertension. Even worse, as many as three quarters of those who have cardiovascular disease along with diabetes can likely attribute it to high blood pressure.

It is not surprising that many of the risk factors for hypertension and cardiovascular disease are the same as for diabetes.

The American Heart Association offers even more information on the connection between cardiovascular disease (CVD) and diabetes:

- 65% of diabetics lose their life to either heart disease or a stroke.

- Diabetics have two to four times the risk of getting heart disease or having a stroke than those who don't have diabetes.

Diabetes is a 100% lifestyle condition caused by eating bread, pastry, cookies, breakfast cereals, pizzas, white rice, high sugar foods, potatoes, parsnips, sugar drinks, and pasta. Diabetes can be controlled to minimize the risk for CVD.

There are critical nutrients missing from the diabetic diet that change the disease outcome when supplemented. Anyone who avoids these unnatural foods and supplements with the missing nutrients does not suffer from diabetes, CVD, and hypertension.

> ▸ *It all starts by choosing a non-inflammatory lifestyle!* ◂

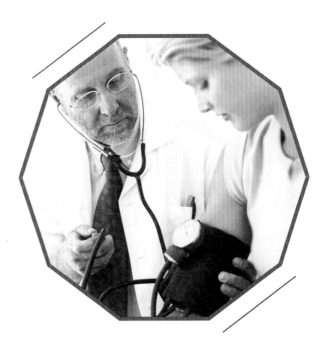

3. Can I Reverse High Blood Pressure?

I do not believe it is appropriate to use the term "cure" for high or low blood pressure since most cases are brought on by lifestyle choices.

Cure is a popular medical buzzword, although the medical field cannot provide cures. (Many people argue that this is on purpose since it would put Big Pharma out of business.) Take away the cause, apply the science of a non-inflammatory lifestyle, and your body will be able to repair itself with a little bit of help. Support tissue regeneration with a healthy lifestyle and the proper nutrients, and in the majority of cases you can become healthy again. If you call that a cure, that's up to you. I prefer to call it living a sensible, healthy lifestyle.

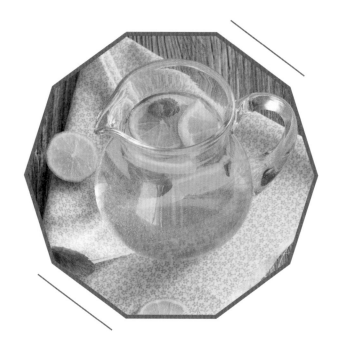

Remember, these conditions are inflammatory in nature and, therefore, will benefit from an anti-inflammatory approach. By hydrating the body with pure, clean water {6-8 x 500 ml (16 oz.) glasses a day} and replenishing it with the proper nutrients and antioxidants in the form of vitamins, minerals, essential fatty acids, healthy carbohydrates, and amino acids, the repair and healing of the body can start to take place.

Nutritional therapy supports healing.

The initial detox can be uncomfortable but only temporarily.

Eating right can minimize the effects.

> ▸ *... regenerate with healthy lifestyle and nutrients ...* ◂

The Genetics

Dr. Caldwell B. Esselstyn Jr., a former surgeon at the Cleveland Clinic, President of the Cleveland Clinic staff, author, and researcher, is famous for saying, "Genes load the gun, but lifestyle pulls the trigger." This is never more applicable than when it comes to high blood pressure.

While genetics can play a role in hypertension, what you choose to do in your everyday life will greatly dictate whether or not your genes will be expressed or activated. For example, most of the risk factors for high blood pressure can be changed through the choices we make.

So, are you doomed to have high blood pressure if it runs in your family?

Absolutely not!

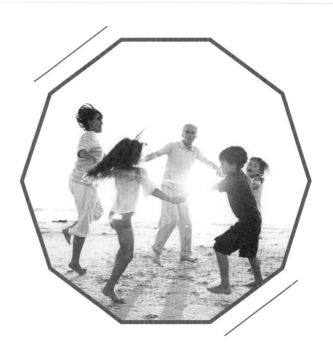

> ▸ *Why are these risk factors so important to be aware of and avoid/minimize?* ◂

As we have already discussed, hypertension is a primary risk factor for cardiovascular disease. When hypertension is left to continue and progress, consequences can be dire.

These consequences include:

- **Damage to the major organs fed by the circulatory system: heart, kidneys, brain, eyes**
- **Coronary heart disease**
- **Left ventricular hypertrophy (thickening of the muscle of the heart's left ventricle)**
- **Stroke**
- **Retinopathy (damaged eyesight)**
- **Kidney disease**
- **Heart failure**

More often than not, hypertension is related to poor lifestyle choices. It can be improved and even "cured" by improving upon these choices.

The Nutrients You Need

Studies show the following nutrients will help prevent or control diabetes in most people:

- **Serrapeptase** - Clears inflammation and scarring.
- **OPC (Grape Seed Extract/ Pycnogen**ol) - Free radical protection, reduces inflammation, promotes healthy blood vessels.
- **Nattokinase** - Enhances the body's natural ability to fight blood clots in several different ways, may also help prevent hardening of the arteries.
- **Curcumin** - Antioxidant, protects and helps tissue healing, scientifically proven to fight inflammation.
- **Ecklonia Cava** - Antioxidant seaweed extract.
- **Vitamin D3 -** Numerous studies show vitamin D3 is critical for immune health and recovery.

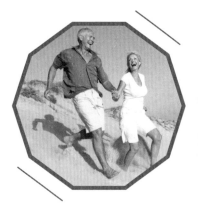

- **Oxygen Promoting Enzymes** - Improve the lungs ability to clear CO2 and take in more oxygen, leading to proper breathing practices.
- **Sodium Thiocyanate/Sodium Hypothiocyanite** - Part of the body's essential defense against infections.
- **Food State Iodine Drops** - Important mineral for immune function.
- **Epicor** - Yeast extract, helps to balance the body's own immune response.
- **Selenium** - Important co-factor of iodine for cell regeneration and protection, facilitates immune function, may lower LDL cholesterol, helps heart muscle regeneration. Contraindicated for some medications.
- **Hempseed** - Essential fatty acid, the king of omegs-3s, simply essential for everyone.
- **GLA (Gamma Linolenic Acid)** - Plant source, essential fatty acid.
- **Alpha-Lipoic Acid R** - Fatty acid, highly effective in reducing inflammation.
- **Digestive Enzymes** - Important when eating cooked foods.

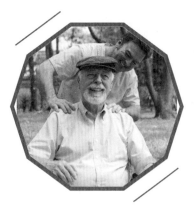

- **Probiotics (Friendly Bacteria)** - To recover gut friendly flora.
- **Multi-Vitamin and Mineral Complex -** To ensure any missing nutrients are covered, especially antioxidants, as together they are protective and slow down artery disease.
- **Natural Vitamin E (D-Alpha- Tocopherol)** - Powerful antioxidant.
- **Vitamin C** - Assists in cardiovascular protection and health.
- **Lycopene** - Decreases risk of cardiovascular disease.
- **Vitamin B Complex** - Increases immune function, converts EFAs into prostaglandins, crucial anti-inflammatory substances.
- **B-6, Folic Acid, B-12** - Essential for lowering homocysteine, a prime marker for heart disease.
- **Potassium** - Precursor to the release of nitric oxide, facilitates sodium excretion, regulates blood pressure.
- **L-Carnitine** - Increases ATP production and boosts energy, allowing regeneration of the heart tissue.
- **Calcium** - Facilitates blood vessel relaxation, reduces blood pressure.

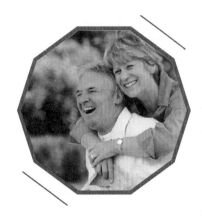

- **Magnesium** - Stabilizes plaque and supports heart rhythm. Assists antioxidants, reduces blood pressure.
- **L-Arginine -** Precursor of nitric oxide, a vasodilator that improves blood flow and the health of the endothelium.
- **D-Ribose -** Quickly restores ATP and energy, allowing regeneration of heart tissue and valves.
- **Manganese -** Facilitates the synthesis of cholesterol and fatty acids.
- **Zinc -** Fights free radicals, facilitates enzyme action.
- ***CoQ10** - Facilitates production of ATP, necessary for energy and a healthy heart muscle.

*Supplementing with CoQ10 is even more critical when taking statin drugs as these drugs inhibit production of CoQ10. Diabetics need to monitor glucose levels closely while taking CoQ10.

4. Why Doesn't My Doctor Tell Me I Can Get Better?

The Non-Inflammatory Lifestyle Program can help you get better! Your doctor is obliged to conform to the drug model that is designed to maintain the monopoly that the pharmaceutical industry, the GMC in the UK and the AMA in the USA, have over all things connected with the health of individuals.

These organizations make profits by caring for sick people and do not have a business model that caters to real healthcare and recovery.

They pursue a patented drug model where they can charge exorbitant prices for a lifetime of drugs that, at best, help individuals feel better and, at worst, speed up their death.

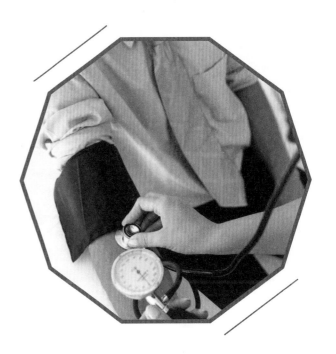

> ▸ *These industries are not designed to get anyone healthy, ever!* ◂

In the USA, they are shielded by the FDA and in the UK by the MHRA. The political parties and the most powerful politicians all receive money from these organizations and are responsible for making the laws that perpetuate this disease management monopoly.

When carefully followed, the Non-Inflammatory Lifestyle Program will show results within 30 days.

5. The Blood Pressure Rehabilitation Plan
Your 10 Steps to a Healthy Future

The following protocol works for any type of blood pressure issue, to some extent.

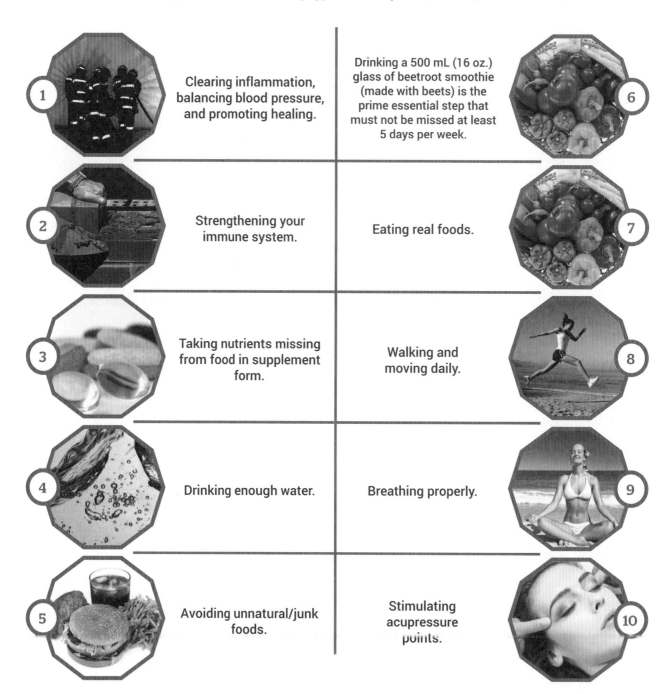

1. Clearing inflammation, balancing blood pressure, and promoting healing.

2. Strengthening your immune system.

3. Taking nutrients missing from food in supplement form.

4. Drinking enough water.

5. Avoiding unnatural/junk foods.

6. Drinking a 500 mL (16 oz.) glass of beetroot smoothie (made with beets) is the prime essential step that must not be missed at least 5 days per week.

7. Eating real foods.

8. Walking and moving daily.

9. Breathing properly.

10. Stimulating acupressure points.

It is almost unheard of for a person applying a good percentage of these lifestyle changes to their daily life to not clear their blood pressure symptoms to some extent, and in many cases completely.

For details of the following suggested formulas, turn to **page 39.**

Clearing Inflammation, Balancing Blood Pressure, and Promoting Healing

#1 Stop Inflammation and Clear Cortisol – **Basic Plan**

RelaxWell™ - To support a relaxed system, lower blood pressure, and reduce anxiety. Take 1 capsule, 3 times a day.

BlockBusterAllClear™ - To support healthy blood flow and circulation. Take 2 capsules, 3 times a day 30 minutes before eating. Drop to 1 x 3 capsules after a month (Plan on 1-2 months).

HealthyFlow - A complete formula to support healthy veins and arteries. Take 4 teaspoons over the day in a little water or juice.

Vitamin D3-K2 Spray - Essential to support normal blood pressure. Take 3 sprays, 2 times per day.

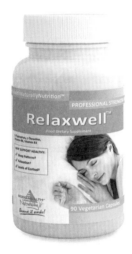 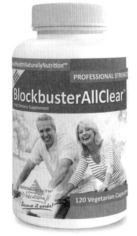 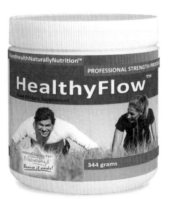 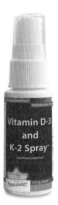

Taking the Missing Nutrients

#2 Blood Pressure Health – **Advanced Plan**

RelaxWell™ - To support a relaxed system, lower blood pressure, and reduce anxiety. Take 1 capsule, 3 times a day.

BlockBusterAllClear™ - To support healthy blood flow and circulation. Take 2 capsules, 3 times a day 30 minutes before eating. Drop to 1 x 3 capsules after a month (Plan on 1-2 months).

HealthyFlow - A complete formula to support healthy veins and arteries. Take 4 teaspoons over the day in a little water or juice.

Vitamin D3-K2 Spray - Essential to support normal blood pressure. Take 3 sprays, 2 times per day.

Ancient Minerals Magnesium OIL ULTRA - To efficiently restore cellular magnesium levels and de-stress the central nervous system. Apply liberally to heart and main limb areas daily.

Nascent Iodine Drops - Important mineral for immune function. Take 4 x 4 drops per day in 25ml of water, swish around the mouth for 30 seconds before swallowing. Build over 2 weeks to 10 x 4 until well and then slowly reduce back to 4 x 4. Note that Iodine needs a supplement containing selenium to activate it such as ActiveLife 90 or Daily Immune Protection.

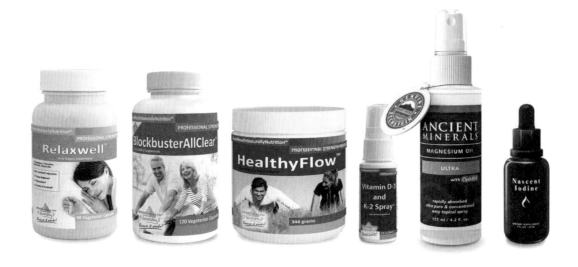

Immune Recovery and Strengthening

#3 Blood Pressure Health – **Ultimate Plan**

RelaxWell™ - To support a relaxed system, lower blood pressure, and reduce anxiety. Take 1 capsule, 3 times a day.

BlockBusterAllClear™ - To support healthy blood flow and circulation. Take 2 capsules, 3 times a day 30 minutes before eating. Drop to 1 x 3 capsules after a month (Plan on 1-2 months).

HealthyFlow - A complete formula to support healthy veins and arteries. Take 4 teaspoons over the day in a little water or juice.

Vitamin D3-K2 Spray - Essential to support normal blood pressure. Take 3 sprays, 2 times per day.

Ancient Minerals Magnesium OIL ULTRA - To efficiently restore cellular magnesium levels and de-stress the central nervous system. Apply liberally to heart and main limb areas daily.

Nascent Iodine Drops - Important mineral for immune function. Take 4 x 4 drops per day in 25ml of water, swish around the mouth for 30 seconds before swallowing. Build over 2 weeks to 10 x 4 until well and then slowly reduce back to 4 x 4. Note that Iodine needs a supplement containing selenium to activate it such as ActiveLife 90 or Daily Immune Protection.

Prescript Assist - World Leading Soil Based Probiotic (the only formula with scientific studies). Take 1 capsule x 2 times a day (can be opened and mixed with food) and then for maintenance at the rate of 1 every 3 days.

Active Life 90 - Powerful Liquid Vitamins & Minerals Formula (300% More Absorbent Than Tablets) Full spectrum multivitamin/mineral with essential selenium, which you should already be taking at 15 ml x 2 times per day with food.

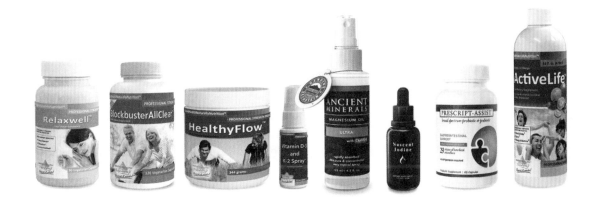

Optional - but suggested for the first 1-2 months at least

A. Ultimate Immune Support Kit
Suggested Formulation
**1st Line (Thiocyanate) Immune
System Support Kit**

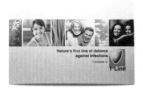

B. Krill Oil
Suggested Formulation
The Krill Miracle

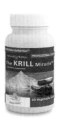

C. Vitamin E Mixed Tocotrienols
Suggested Formulation:
Naturally Better Vitamin E

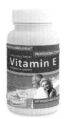

D. Digestive Enzymes
Suggested Formulation:
Essential Digestive Plus™

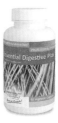

4. Drinking enough water.

Drink 6-8 glasses of distilled or RO filtered water per day, with a large pinch of bicarbonate of soda (baking soda).

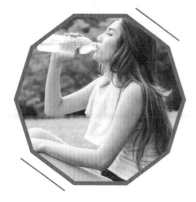

5. Avoiding eating unnatural junk foods.

Until completely recovered, stop eating all starchy carbohydrates (breads, pastry, cookies, breakfast cereals, potatoes, and pasta), processed foods, and milk products.

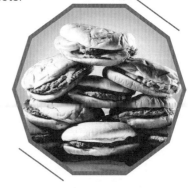

Note: Do not eat: potatoes, parsnips, turnips, and rice (except for small amount of wild or brown rice and yams/sweet potatoes).

6. Drinking a 500ml (16 oz.) Glass of Beetroot Smoothie (Made with Beets) Is the Prime Essential Step That Must Not Be Missed At Least 5 Days per Week

Studies show that eating two beets (beetroots) in a smoothie, soup, or salad every day will reduce high blood pressure within hours and increase stamina. Every day or at least every other day is best to maintain this benefit. Breakfast is the best time.

Example: Beetroot Smoothie with Carrot and Celery

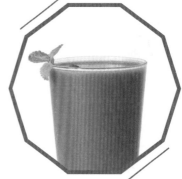

- 2 small beetroots (the smaller, the sweeter)
- 2 large carrots
- 1 stalk of celery
- 1 apple
- Ginger to taste

7. Eating Really Healthy Foods

**Include some of the following foods every 2 hours for the first few months:

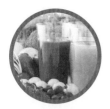

Eat 9-14 portions of fresh or frozen veggies daily (in soups, juiced, stir-fries, steamed, etc.); 50% raw juiced (use the pulp in soups) and organic if possible. Blended makes for better digestion.

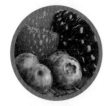

Eat 5 portions of antioxidant rich, dark skinned fruits (blueberries, cherries, red grapes, etc.) daily.

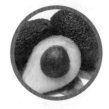

Avocados are the all-time super food with nearly a full spectrum of nutrients. If they are available where you live, make sure you have at least 2 per day for good health recovery. All blood pressure issues (as well as cancer and heart disease) are helped by these.

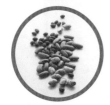

Eat 5 portions of beans, nuts, and seeds (soaked and mashed for the nuts and seeds).

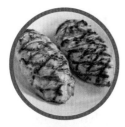

If you want to eat meat, then choose pasture-fed meats or chicken and eat only a small amount weekly. Grass-fed is healthier than grain or corn-fed animals.

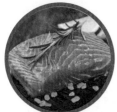

If you eat fish, then eat at least 3-4 portions per week of oily fish and vary it by choosing fish such as salmon, sardines, mackerel, etc. Even canned fish is very nutritious, and wild caught fish is best.

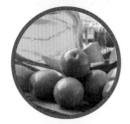

Include Hemp, Omega 3, or Krill oil and other healthy oils like Olive oil and Coconut oil.

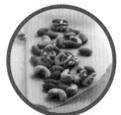

As healthy alternatives to carbs, consider Quinoa, Chia Seeds, Amaranth, Buckwheat, and Millet Seeds. Cous Cous can be used, except for those who are allergic to gluten proteins (celiacs, etc.).

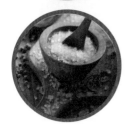

Take 3-5 (depending upon your body mass and the heat) teaspoons of Sea or Rock Salt daily in food or a little water. Sea or Rock Salt does not contain the critical mineral iodine so add Nascent Iodine to your daily dose.

▶ *A potassium-rich diet is essential for everyone and especially for those with blood pressure issues.* ◀

Have at least 4 of these potassium-rich foods per day:

- 1 avocado - 975 mg
- 1 banana - 422 mg
- 1 cup of mushroom - 428 mg
- 1 salmon fillet (frozen wild is best) - 534 mg
- 1/2 cup of dried apricots (snack over the day) - 725 mg
- 1 cup cooked spinach - 839 mg
- 1 cup bean (adzuki, white, lima) - 1004 mg

Recommended Vegetables

Note: Vegetables may not be available in all countries.

- Artichoke
- Asian Vegetables Sprouts (Wheat, Barley, Alfalfa, etc)
- Asparagus
- Avocado
- Broad Beans
- Cabbage (various types)
- Dandelion Leaves
- Dried Peas
- Fennel
- Garden Peas
- Garlic
- Kale
- Lettuce (Kos and various types)
- Mangetout Peas
- Mushrooms
- Petit Pois Peas
- Runner Beans
- Seaweed all types (Kelp, Wakame, Noni, etc)
- Sugar Snap Peas
- Beetroot
- Broccoli
- Brussel Sprouts
- Capsicum
- Carrots
- Cauliflower
- Celeriac
- Choko
- Cucumber
- Eggplant (Aubergine) Kale
- Kohlrabi
- Kumara
- Okra
- Onions (Red and White)
- Radishes
- Silver Beet
- Spinach
- Squash
- Zucchini (Courgettes)

Recommended Fruits

Note: Fruits may not be available in all countries.

- Apple
- Apricot
- Avocado
- Blackberries
- Blackcurrants
- Bilberries
- Blueberries
- Cherries
- Cherimoya
- Dates
- Damsons
- Durian
- Figs
- Gooseberries
- Grapes
- Grapefruit
- Kiwi fruit
- Limes
- Lychees
- Mango
- Nectarine
- Orange
- Pear
- Plum/Prune (dried Plum)
- Pineapple
- Pomegranate
- Raspberries
- Western raspberry (blackcap)
- Rambutan
- Salal berry
- Satsuma
- Strawberries
- Tangerine

The Garden of Eden Pyramid

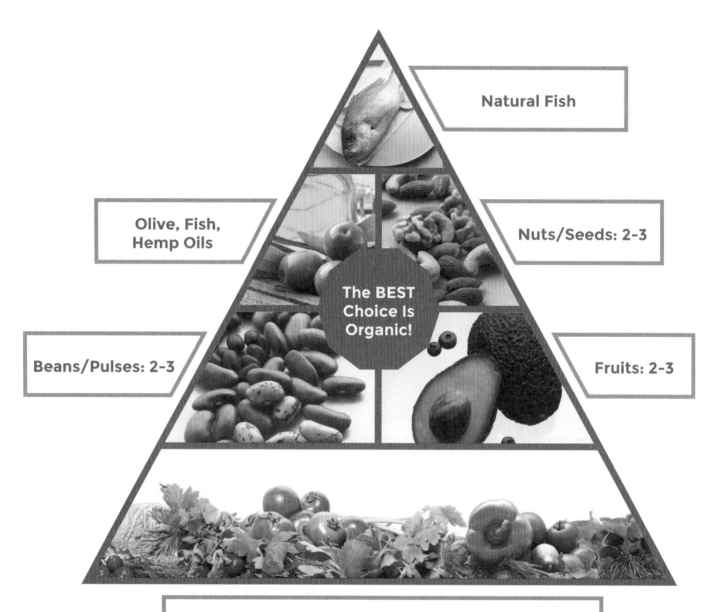

Natural Fish

Olive, Fish, Hemp Oils

Nuts/Seeds: 2-3

The BEST Choice Is Organic!

Beans/Pulses: 2-3

Fruits: 2-3

Vegetables (excluding root): 8-12 servings a day
1/2 raw veggies: salads, etc.

8. Walking and Moving Daily

Contrary to the opinion of fitness fanatics, there are two simple ways to get your body working better and stronger. And no, they do not include swimming and cycling, although you can add these later if you want to.

▶ *One of the two simple ways to exercise is to build up to walking 3-5 miles per day, in a fast, purposely strong way with as long a stride as you can. Keep your hands moving from chest level to belt level as you move with each stride.*

Use weights or wrist weights as you improve.

If this is difficult for you at the start, and your lungs are weak, then lie down to exercise to make it easier. ◀

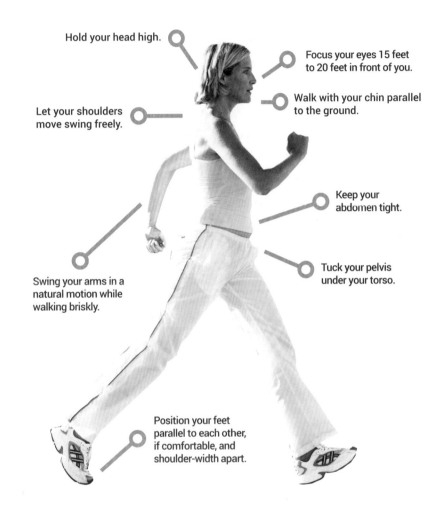

Hold your head high.

Focus your eyes 15 feet to 20 feet in front of you.

Walk with your chin parallel to the ground.

Let your shoulders move swing freely.

Keep your abdomen tight.

Tuck your pelvis under your torso.

Swing your arms in a natural motion while walking briskly.

Position your feet parallel to each other, if comfortable, and shoulder-width apart.

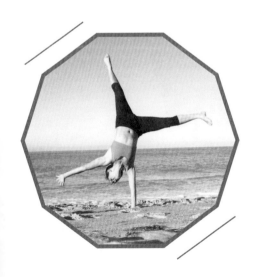

Lie down in a comfortable place. On your bed, (if it's firm enough), when you first wake up is a great time and place for this. Bring a knee up to your chest as high as you can get it and then alternate with the other knee. Do as many of these as you can while keeping count. Do this every day and set yourself targets to increase the speed and the number as the weeks go by. You should be doing enough to make your lungs and heart beat faster. At the same time, as you improve your count on your back you need to be starting your walking and building this up.

The second great exercise for strengthening your lungs is to build up slowly where you can exercise at maximum rate for 2 minutes, 6 times per day. It does not matter what exercise you do, e.g. skipping, star jumps, running on the spot; just about anything, as long as your heart and lungs are working at maximum capacity. By working at maximum rate, your lungs and muscles connected with your heart and lungs will get stronger.

Physical activity is vital to your rehabilitation plan.

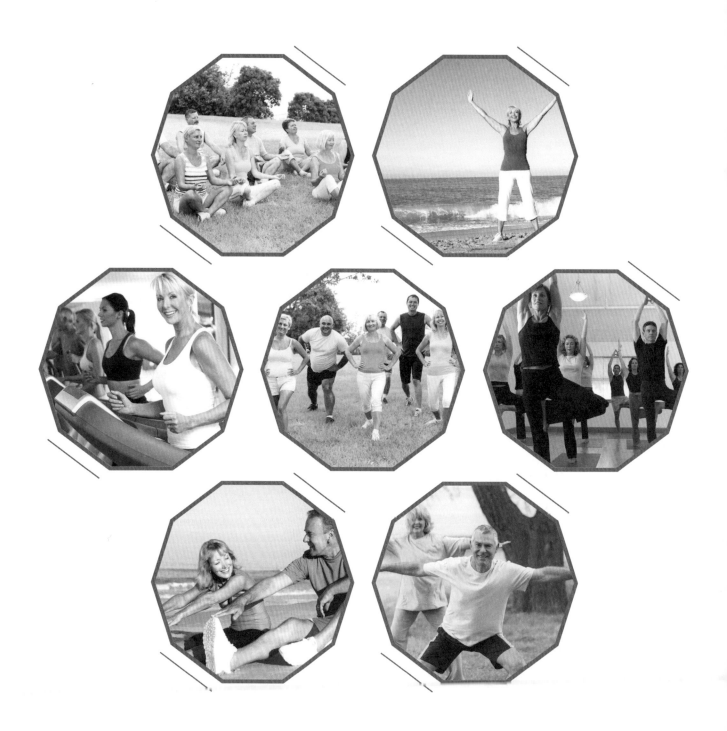

9. Breathing Properly

It is critical to breathe properly, especially to improve circulation. There are two ways to breathe. The first one is an anxious breath in the chest, and the second is a relaxed breath in the diaphragm, or more precisely, in the tummy area.

The first breath in the chest is part of the stress response and involves hormones such as cortisol. This type of breathing should last no longer than it takes to deal with a problem in life and then another hormone kicks in to create relaxed breathing. If this stress type of breathing becomes chronic or habitual, then the cortisol and retained carbon dioxide become part of the problem, and the body's natural healthy systems cannot function properly. It also weakens the immune system and opens you up to infections.

Your goal is to relearn relaxed, healthy breathing, where you clear cortisol and carbon dioxide. Too much carbon dioxide in your bloodstream destroys something called hemoglobin, which is the blood's method of carrying oxygen around the body. So it's critical to be able to breathe in a relaxed way from the diaphragm.

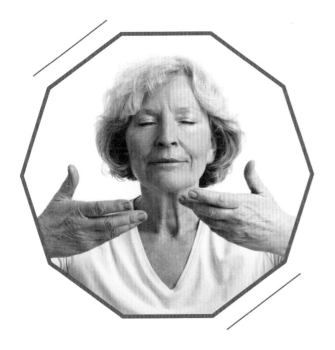

HOW TO BREATHE PROPERLY

The simple way to learn is to lie on your back in a firm bed or on the floor on a blanket or mat. Put a bit of weight over your belly button, such as a heavy book. Take a breath into your nose so that the book rises as you fill your diaphragm (tummy) with air. Hold the breath in your tummy for the count of 4 and then breathe out through your nose and feel your tummy deflating. Let go of any tension you may have with the out-breath. Then repeat. Your upper chest should not move at all, which shows you are relaxed and not stress breathing.

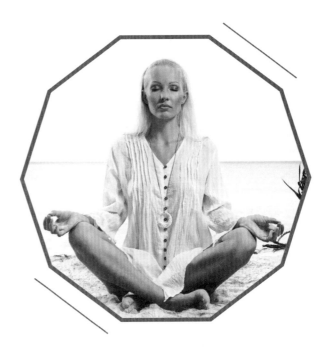

▶ *Practice over and again while lying down, and once you have really got the long, slow rhythm of relaxed breathing, then try it standing up. You may feel dizzy to begin with getting all this fresh oxygen, but you must practice this every spare minute you have.*

Measure your BP before and after breathing exercises and see the difference yourself. ◀

Meditation to Reduce Stress

Research supports meditation as a stress-reduction technique to benefit the health of the heart. One study that tracked 200 patients over five years showed that those who practiced meditation greatly reduced their risk of heart attack, stroke, and death by close to 50% compared to patients who didn't meditate. *(Medical College of Wisconsin in collaboration with the Institute for Natural Medicine and Prevention)*

The group of patients that meditated also had benefits like:

- Remaining disease-free for a longer period of time.
- Reduced blood pressure.
- Lower levels of stress.

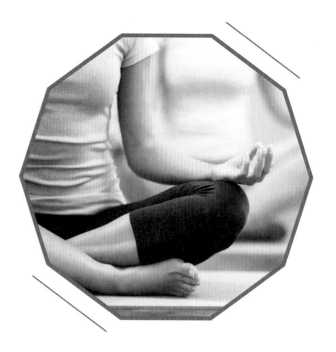

Why is meditation so beneficial for a healthy heart? Regular meditation can help to alleviate stress. As a result, this will lower levels of the stress hormone cortisol and calm inflammatory processes in the body that can lead to hardened arteries and atherosclerosis.

Recommendations: Calm your mind with meditation using a guided meditation CD or sitting in silence for just 5 minutes a day. Increase your meditation sessions over time.

> ▸ *As research confirms, stress reduction can work wonders to boost the health of the heart.* ◂

The health of your heart may also depend on a mind-body connection, in cooperation with a healthy, noninflammatory lifestyle. Consider holistic activities like:

Yoga

Yoga can improve flexibility, mindfulness, mood, and sleep. Yoga can also improve heart rate variability, an indicator of a healthy heart. One Ohio State University study showed that women that regularly practiced yoga had lower cytokine interleukin-6 (IL-6) levels, which contribute to the inflammatory response in the body and have been linked with heart disease, stroke, arthritis, type 2 diabetes, and a number of other chronic diseases.

Recommendations: Try 20 minutes of yoga, 3 days a week to support heart health.

Pilates

Pilates is known to improve flexibility, posture, and core strength to remedy lower back pain. It can also support heart fitness. According to the American College of Sports Medicine, intermediate Pilates is equivalent to walking at 4-4.5 mph on a treadmill; advanced Pilates is equivalent to a moderate-high intensity workout. All Pilates practices will improve circulation.

Recommendations: Try a 10 to 20 minute Pilates workout, 3 days a week to support heart health.

Tai Chi

Tai Chi is a form of moving meditation that uses mental concentration and controlled motion to challenge the body. Tai Chi also provides health benefits to reduce blood pressure and stress and boost the health of the heart. A BMC Complementary and Alternative Medicine review confirms that Tai Chi can decrease anxiety, depression, and stress, while improving self-esteem.

Recommendations: Try one or more Tai Chi classes a week under the guidance of an instructor to support heart health.

Practicing at least one of these mind-body techniques can greatly contribute to the health of your heart and serve as a vital component in your Blood Pressure Rehabilitation Program.

> *▸ Stress reduction and heart health go hand-in-hand! ◂*

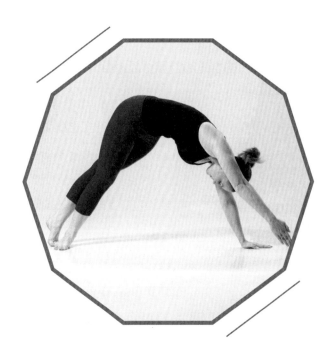

10. Stimulating the Acupressure Points

The fastest way to lower (or raise) your blood pressure is by stimulating acupressure points. There are various points, which you can massage gently with your finger or stimulate with an electronic stimulator that mimics the action of acupuncture. The recommended device is **HealthPoint™**, and you can read more about this on **page 48**.

BONUS: Getting Out into the Sun As Much As Possible

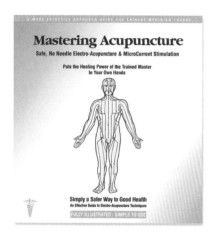

A critical vitamin for healthy blood pressure is Vitamin D3. There is a large dose of this in the important supplement I recommend on **page 41**, but it is still essential to still get some Vitamin D from the sun.

The sun is the bringer of all life, and a silly myth has developed that the sun is our enemy and we should keep out of it, or worse still, put some toxic chemicals all over us so we can go out in it.

I am not saying that we can go out on a really hot sunny day and lie in the sun for 6 hours for the first time. We are supposed to build the skin's tolerance to the sun over many weeks in the spring to stimulate protection from it, so that by the time the hot summer sun comes along we can tolerate much more.

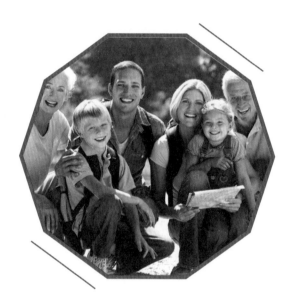

Recommendations:

A. Get as much skin exposed to the sun as you can every day, e.g. on your daily walk.

B. Build up slowly from the spring to summer time.

C. Try not to stay out in the middle of the day without covering up, and cover up rather than use a barrier cream.

D. If you do use a sun cream, get an organic one rather than chemical ones with well-known names.

E. Remember, the sun is your friend, and as with friends, try not to get too much in one go!

More About Clearing Inflammation, Balancing Blood Pressure, and Promoting Healing

RelaxWell™ is a special formula created from tried and true quality ingredients known to support more restful and healthy sleep patterns with a combination of B-Vitamins to act as powerful aids against high stress and unwieldy cortisol levels.

> ▸ *RelaxWell™ combines L-Tryptophan, L-Theanine, Vitamin B6, and Vitamin B3 to make for a much better rested YOU!* ◂

L-Tryptophan is an essential amino acid and the precursor to serotonin. Serotonin is a neurotransmitter responsible for transmitting nerve impulses in the brain, inducing sleep and tranquility, and stabilizing function of the central nervous system. Serotonin deficiencies, which are related to L-Tryptophan deficiencies, are well documented in cases of depression and insomnia.

L-Theanine is a natural phytochemical found in Japanese green tea. L-Theanine is a non-essential amino acid that is present in the brain and is a close relative of Glutamate. Studies indicate that L-Theanine interacts with the neurotransmitter GABA (gamma-aminobutyrate). GABA, known for its importance in nervous system functioning, works with the mood centers of the brain.

RelaxWell™ - Suitable for Vegetarians and Vegans

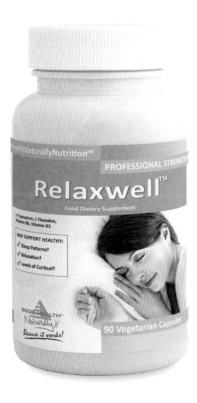

Active Ingredients:

L-TRYPTOPHAN (500mg)

L-THEANINE (100mg)

50% of your daily value of VITAMIN B3 - NICOTINIC ACID (10mg)

50% of your daily value of VITAMIN B3 - NIACINAMIDE (10mg)

500% of your daily value of VITAMIN B6 - PYRIDOXINE HCl (10mg)

Other Ingredients:

Maltodextrin
Microcrystalline Cellulose
Magnesium Stearate

Dosage:

Take 1 capsule, 3 times a day.

BlockBusterAllClear™ is, by any measure, the best and most powerful enzyme formula available. The careful blend of powerful enzymes such as Serrapeptase, Nattokinase, Digestive Enzyme, antioxidants and proanthocyanidins such as Grape Seed Extract and Pycnogenol now in a delayed release capsule - all with a long history of studies and a reputation for great effect - means this is perfect for those requiring the highest level of support for their health or just long term maintenance.

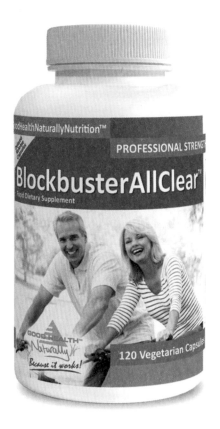

Benefits include:

- Help for discomfort in your legs and veins.
- Revitalization of your cardiovascular and arterial system.
- Nutrients for healthy joints and cartilage.
- Nutrients for wound and trauma healing.
- Healthier aging and lower inflammation.

Ingredients:

Serrapeptase 80,000 IU
Nattokinase* 1600 FU
Protease 20,000 HUT
Lipase 1500 FIP
Amylase 4000 DU
Cellulase 600 CU
Lactase 1000 ALU
Acerola extract 50 mg
Amla extract 50 mg
Olive Leaf Citrus Blend 230 mg
Trace Minerals (Coral Calcium) 100 mg
Bacillus Coagulans 376,000,000 CFU
Protease S 5 mg
Grapeseed extract 100 mg
Policosanol 6 mg
Pycnogenol® 10 mg

Dosage:

Take 2 x 3 times per day, 30 mins before eating and drop to 1 x 3 after 1 month (plan on 1-2 months)

HealthyFlow™ contains L-Arginine, a protein amino acid present in the proteins of all life forms. It is classified as a semi-essential or conditionally essential amino acid. This means that under normal circumstances the body can synthesize sufficient L-Arginine to meet physiological demands. There are, however, conditions where the body cannot. L-Arginine is a precursor in the formation of Nitric Oxide, Creatine, Polyamines, L-Glutamate, L-Proline, Agmatin (a possible neurotransmitter in the brain) and the Arginine-containing Tetrapeptide Tuftsin, believed to be an immunomodulator.

Vitamin D3/Vitamin K2 spray for protecting your heart against cardiovascular disease. Vitamin D3/ K2 boosts a protein called MGP, which protects blood vessels against calcification.

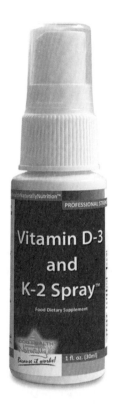

Amazing benefits are shown in studies, like:

- Healthy Blood Flow
- Healthy Cardio System
- Healthy Blood Pressure
- Healthy Male Fertility
- Healthy Kidneys

Ingredients:

L-Arginine- 5.000mg
L-Lysine- 1,500mg
L-Citrulline - 200 mg
Grapeseed Extract 95% - 150 mg
AstraGin™ (contains Astraglaus membrenaceus and Panax notoginseng) - 50 mg
Grape Skin Extract 4:1 (Polyphenols) - 25 mg
Proprietary Blend (Citric Acid, BeFlora, Potassium Sorbate, Silica) - 3840 mg

Dosage:

Take 4 teaspoons over the day in a little water or juice.

Ingredients:

Vitamin D3 – 1000IU
Vitamin K2 MK7 – 100mcg

Dosage:

Take 3 sprays, 2 times per day.

More About Missing Nutrients

Ancient Minerals Magnesium Oil Ultra is a next generation formula incorporating the unique synergistic benefits of MSM and magnesium. Ancient Minerals Magnesium Oil Ultra offers improved uptake of magnesium ions and enhanced cell membrane permeability; it can be used for pain management, joint mobility, and calming inflammation.

Nascent Iodine is totally different from the typical iodine in its denser state sold as an antiseptic, or as iodine tri-chloride (claiming to be atomized), or as added to potassium iodide to make it soluble in liquid. Nascent Iodine is a consumable iodine in its atomic form rather than its molecular form. It can provide benefits in thyroid and immune support, detoxification, metabolism, improved energy, and more.

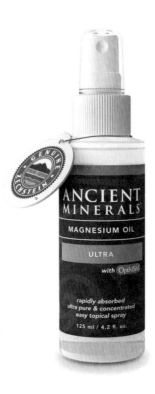

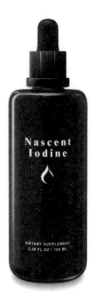

Ingredients:

Iodine (in its atomic form) 400 µg

Dosage:

Take 4 x 4 drops per day in 25ml of water, swish around the mouth for 30 seconds before swallowing. Build over 2 weeks to 10 x 4 until well and then slowly reduce back to 4 x 4. Note that Iodine needs a supplement containing selenium to activate it such as ActiveLife 90 or Daily Immune Protection.

Ingredients:

1.6g elemental magnesium per fl oz.
3.6g of MSM (OptiMSM®) per fl oz.

Dosage:

Apply to heart and chest muscles, large limb muscles, and neck muscles daily after showering.

More About Immune Strengthening Formulations

Prescript-Assist®️ (P-A) is a 3rd-generation combination of 29 probiotic microflora "Soil-Based- Organisms (SBOs)" uniquely combined with a humic/ fulvic acid prebiotic that enhances SBO proliferation. Prescript-Assist's®️ microflora are Class-1 micro ecological units that are typical of those progressively found resident along the healthy human GI tract.

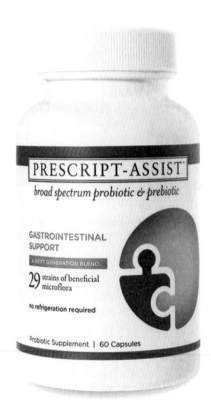

Ingredients:

Proprietary blend of Leonardite

Class I (beneficial microorganisms): Anthrobacter agilis, Anthrobacter citreus, Anthrobacter globiformis, Anthrobacter luteus, Anthrobacter simplex, Acinetobacter calcoaceticus, Azotobacter chroococcum, Azotobacter paspali, Azospirillum brasiliense, Azospirillum lipoferum, Bacillus brevis, Bacillus marcerans, Bacillus pumilis, Bacillus polymyxa, Bacillus subtilis, Bacteroides lipolyticum, Bacteriodes succinogenes, Brevibacterium lipolyticum, Brevibacterium stationis, Kurtha zopfil, Myrothecium verrucaria, Pseudomonas calcis, Pseudomonas dentrificans, Pseudomonas flourescens, Pseudomonas glathei, Phanerochaete chrysosporium, Streptomyces fradiae, Streptomyces celluslosae, Streptomyces griseoflavus

Dosage:

Take 1 capsule x 2 times a day (can be opened and mixed with food) and then for maintenance at the rate of 1 every 3 days.

Active Life 90 Powerful Liquid Vitamins & Minerals is a liquid formula to ensure you get all the essential vitamins and minerals needed by your body. This single liquid supplement allows for maximum absorption and utilization of the body - 300% more absorbent than tablets!

Ingredients	Amount per Serving
• Calories	39
• Calcium (Tricalcium Phosphate, Citrate)	600mg
• Choline Bitartrate	25mg
• Chromium (Chromium Polynicotinate)	200mcg
• Copper (Copper Gluconate)	2mg
• Folic Acid (Vitamin B Conjugate)	500mcg
• Inositol	50mg
• Magnesium (Citrate Gluconate Concentrate)	300mg
• Manganese (Manganese Gluconate)	10mg
• Organic Seleniumethionine	200mcg
• Potassium (Potassium Gluconate)	250mg
• Vitamin A (Palmitate)	5000IU
• Vitamin A (Beta Carotene)	5000IU
• Vitamin B1 (Thiamine Mononitrate)	3mg
• Vitamin B12 (Methylcobalamin)	6mcg
• Vitamin B2 (Riboflavin)	3.4mg
• Vitamin B3 (Niacinamide)	40mg
• Vitamin B5 (Calcium Pantothenate)	20mg
• Vitamin B6 (Pyridoxine Hydrochloride)	4mg
• Vitamin C (Ascorbic Acid)	300mg
• Vitamin D (Cholecalciferol)	400IU
• Vitamin E (Alpha Tocopheryl Acetate)	60IU
• Vitamin K (Phytonadione)	80mcg
• Zinc (Oxide)	15mg
• Ionic Trace Minerals	600mg
• Phosphorus (Amino Acid Chelate)	190mg
• Biotin	300mcg
• Iodine (Potassium Iodine)	150mcg
• Boron (Sodium Borate)	2mg
• Molybdenum	75mcg
• Chloride Concentrate	102mg
• Amino Acid Complex	10mg
• Aloe Vera Extract (200:1)	2 mg

Dosage:

Take 15ml x 2 times daily with meals.

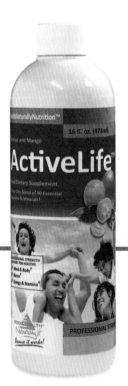

More About Optional Nutrients

1st Line (Thiocyanate) Immune System Support Kit

1st Line is a new all natural product to fight against many types of infections including viruses. It is a patented formula by a British Chemist containing Thiocyanate Ions. When added to water 1st Line provides a drink which forms the same molecules that make up our body's first line of defence against all types of bacteria, yeast, fungi, flu, germs and viruses. 1st Line offers the aggressive attack to these unwanted infections without doing harm to healthy bacteria in the body, a common side-effect when using antibiotic drugs. 1st line is safe and easy to use.

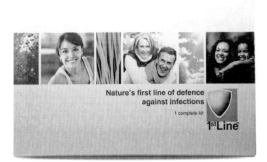

Ingredients:

Sodium Thiocyanate 100ppm
Sodium Hypothiocyanate 60ppm

Dosage:

Take 1 kit daily for 3 days (total of 3). 1st Line Kit should always be taken at least 90 minutes before and after food, approximately. 3 kits are the minimum and in serious conditions 10 kits over 10 days are better if finances allow.

Antarctic Pure Krill Oil

Krill are tiny shrimp-like crustaceans found in the Southern Oceans. The Southern Oceans are the only oceans in the world that remain unpolluted by the heavy toxic metals that are now found in many fish oils. Krill are a super rich source of Omega 3, 6, and 9, and their antioxidant levels are 300 times greater than Vitamins A and E and 48 times greater than Omega 3 found in standard fish oils. (Please note: People with seafood allergies should notify their physician prior to taking a Krill or fish dietary supplement.)

The unique combination of antioxidants, Omega 3, 6, and 9 oils and other potent ingredients in 100% natural Neptune-source Antarctic Pure Krill Oil offers support for:

*   **A reduction in lung/heart-damaging inflammation**
*   **Improved concentration, memory, and learning**
*   **Improvement in cholesterol and other blood lipid levels**
*   **Stabilization of blood sugar levels**
*   **Healthy joints, with a decrease in pain and symptoms associated with arthritis**
*   **Fighting the damaging effects of aging**
*   **Protecting cell membranes**
*   **Healthy liver function**
*   **Bolstering the immune system**
*   **Healthy mood regulation**
*   **Optimal skin health**
*   **Improved quality of life**

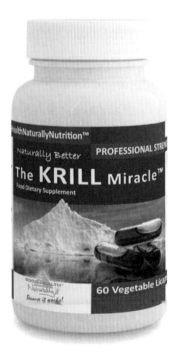

Ingredients:

Superba™ Krill Oil - 1000mg
Phospholipids - 450mg
Total Omega 3 - 250mg
EPA - 120mg
DHA - 70mg
Omega 6 - 15mg
Omega 9 - 80mg
Astaxanthin - 110µg

Dosage:

Take 1 capsule twice per day with food.

Naturally Better Vitamin E

Offers a self-emulsifying delivery system that provides a consistent oral absorption of Tocotrienols. It can provide support for hair growth, Alzheimer's disease, stroke-induced injuries, non-alcoholic fatty liver disease, cardio-protection, cholesterol reduction, immune function, and especially cystic fibrosis.

Essential Digestive Plus™

The digestive system is a truly integrated system – the function of one aspect usually affects the other. Because of this interrelationship among the components of the digestive system, it is often difficult to determine the exact cause of any digestive disturbance. However, using the proper digestive enzymes can eliminate most of the problems.

Incomplete digestion and yeast can be the main contributors to the development of many diseases. Ingesting foods and nutritional supplements are of little benefit if their break down and assimilation are inadequate, but supplementing with enzymes helps allow for better absorption.

Proper small intestine absorption requires effective digestive enzymes coupled with fully functional absorptive surfaces. Improving small intestine function includes addressing the underlying issues that cause the discomfort and disease. Digestive enzymes can help bring relief to food intolerance and allergies, and provide support when the body is suffering from a lack of enzymes, low immune status, and too much sugar in the diet.

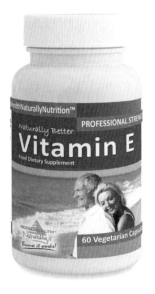
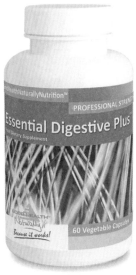

Ingredients:

FrutaFit® Inulin   150mg
Protease   82,000HUT
Amylase   8,000IU
Lipase   1,350FIP
Alpha Galactosidase   300 GLA
Invertase   525INVU
Lactase   1,000ALU
Pectinase   55endoPGU
Glucoamylase   20AGU
Cellulase   600CU

Ingredients:

Total d-Mixed-Tocotrienols and Tocopherols (Tocomin*) 20.00 mg
Vitamin E Activity, IU 8.06 IU
Plant Squalene 4.92 mg
Phytosterol 1.72 mg

Dosage:

Take 1 capsule, 2 times per day.

Dosage:

Take 1 capsule as you start your meals, 3 times per day.

More About Acupressure

Stimulating the angina and palpitation points on pages 3.4 and 3.5 of the book **Mastering Acupuncture** will help to balance the heart/circulatory system. These points can be effectively and safely stimulated using the **HealthPoint**™ electro-acupressure kit. The advantage of the kit is it gives you the power to precisely locate the acupuncture point, and indeed other points, so you can enjoy the benefits of acupuncture at home and without any needles.

HealthPoint™ is easy to use, painless, and effective. It includes an instructional DVD and book covering over 150 pain and non-pain conditions that can be helped, such as headaches, back, neck, and joint problems.

The gentle and systematic stimulation of the body's natural healing system can speed recovery in many cases. **HealthPoint**™ breakthrough technology was developed by leading pain control specialist Dr. Julian Kenyon MD 21 years ago, and today features the latest microchip technology to quickly locate acupuncture points key to specific health conditions, such as the points for High Blood Pressure and Low Blood Pressure.

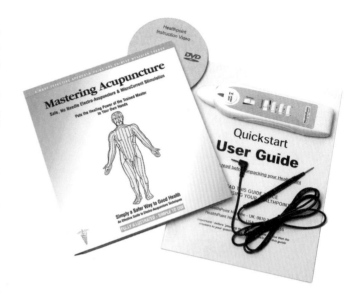

In Conclusion:

The Non-Inflammatory Lifestyle Program is a complete program, one designed to address all aspects of what is required to eliminate hypertension:

- A treatment structured for those patients struggling to obtain healthy blood pressure, even after other medical treatments have failed.
- A program that can help you learn how to love your new lifestyle and improve your quality of life.
- A rehabilitation plan that includes treatment in the form of exercise, education, and coaching.
- A personalized program that incorporates therapy and support, assisting you in achieving the maximum results possible.

High blood pressure is essentially a lifestyle condition, meaning if the lifestyle is changed, there is every likelihood of some recovery. With the changes in this 10 Step Plan put into effect, the body is perfectly capable of healing and recovering good health.

▸ *Drugs don't make you healthy.* ◂

Drugs do not work in that they do not make you healthy. At best, drugs will help you feel better; at worst, they will speed up degeneration and contribute to premature death.

The pharmaceutical business would prefer you continue your present, ineffective treatment plan, only utilizing toxic pills in the form of immune-suppressing drugs and avoiding the true path to prevention and healing.

▸ *You are now learning there is a better way.* ◂

The Non-Inflammatory Lifestyle Program is detailed within this book and, when carefully followed, will show results within weeks.

▸ *You will always end up healthier with this plan.* ◂

The worst thing that can happen with this plan is that you will get healthier but still need to take drugs if they or the disease have damaged you to the extent that you are reliant on them.

▸ *Take it all slowly and step by step.* ◂

Unless you are already used to making changes in your life, you will find adopting these habits of healthy living can be difficult to sustain. Persist. Because...

▸ *Make no mistake... Your life is worth it.* ◂

Robert Redfern, Your Health Coach

Email robert@goodhealth.nu
www.MyGoodHealthClub.com
for step by step coaching and support.

Sample Daily Blood Pressure Plan

TIME	ACTION	AMOUNT
BREAKFAST		
After your daily shower	Ancient Minerals Magnesium Oil Ultra with OptiMSM	Apply to heart and main limb areas daily
Before Breakfast	HealthPoint Kit	Use daily on appropriate Microcurrent stimulation points as necessary
Before Breakfast	1st Line Kit	Take 1 kit daily
Before Breakfast	Relaxwell	Take 1 capsule
Before Breakfast	BlockBuster AllClear	Take 2 capsules
Before Breakfast	HealthyFlow	Take 2 teaspoons in a little water or juice
Before Breakfast	Vitamin D3/K2 Spray	Take 3 sprays
Before Breakfast	Nascent Iodine	Take 4 drops in 25ml of water
Before Breakfast	Prescript-Assist	Take 1 capsule
Before Breakfast	ActiveLife 90	Take 15ml with a little juice or water
Before Breakfast	The Krill Miracle/Hemp Seed Oil	Take 1 capsule/ 1 teaspoon
Before Breakfast	B4 Health Spray	Take 4 sprays
Before Breakfast	Essential Digestive Plus	Take 1 capsule x 3 times a day
LUNCH		
Before Lunch	Relaxwell	Take 1 capsule
Before Lunch	BlockBuster AllClear	Take 2 capsules
Lunch	HealthyFlow	Take 2 teaspoons in a little water or juice
Lunch	Vitamin D3/K2 Spray	Take 3 sprays
Lunch	Essential Digestive Plus	Take 1 capsule
Lunch	Nascent Iodine	Take 4 drops in 25ml of water
Lunch	Ubiquinol	Take 2 capsules with food
Lunch	Vitamin E	Take 1 capsule
BREAK		
Break	Nascent Iodine	Take 4 drops in 25ml of water
EVENING MEAL		
Before Dinner	Relaxwell	Take 1 capsule
Before Dinner	BlockBuster AllClear	Take 2 capsules
Dinner	Nascent Iodine	Take 4 drops in 25ml of water
Dinner	ActiveLife™ 90 Vitamins/Minerals	Take 15ml with juice or water
Dinner	The Krill Miracle/Hemp Seed Oil	Take 1 capsule/1 teaspoon
Dinner	Prescript-Assist	Take 1 capsule
Dinner	Vitamin E	Take 1 capsule
Dinner	Essential Digestive Plus	Take 1 capsule

All the books in the Heart and Cardiovascular Series:

- Angina Cardiomyopathy
- Diseased Valves
- DVT
- Coronary Heart
- Stroke Recovery
- Carotid Arteries/Arterial Vascular Diseases
- Thrombosis
- Atrial Fibrillation Palpitations
- Heart Failure
- CVD
- Blood Pressure

Other Books by Robert Redfern:

- The 'Miracle Enzyme' is Serrapeptase
- Turning A Blind Eye
- Mastering Acupuncture
- EquiHealth Equine acupressure